DASH YOUR WAY TO HEALTH

A Comprehensive Guide to the Diet and Exercise Program that Lowers Blood Pressure and Promotes Weight Loss.

Disclaimer

TABLE OF CONTENTS

INTRODUCTION

What is the DASH Diet and Exercise Program, and Why Do You Need It?

Are you looking for a simple, effective, and enjoyable way to improve your health and well-being? Do you want to lower your blood pressure, lose weight, and enhance your metabolism and mood? Do you want to prevent or manage chronic diseases such as cardiovascular disease, stroke, diabetes, and kidney disease? You're in the right place if you said "yes" to any of these questions. This book will introduce you to the DASH diet and exercise program, a comprehensive and holistic approach to achieving your health and fitness goals.

The DASH diet and exercise program is based on the Dietary Approaches to Stop Hypertension (DASH) study, a landmark research project that was conducted by the National Institutes of Health in the 1990s. The study found that a diet rich in fruits, vegetables, whole grains, low-fat dairy, lean protein, nuts, seeds, and legumes, and low in salt, saturated fat, cholesterol, and sugar, can significantly lower blood pressure and reduce the risk of cardiovascular disease, stroke, diabetes, and kidney disease. The study also found that combining the DASH diet with moderate physical activity can enhance the benefits of the diet and improve overall fitness and well-being.

The DASH diet and exercise program are not a fad or a quick fix. It is a lifestyle change that requires commitment, consistency, and patience. But it is also a lifestyle change that is easy to follow, flexible to adapt to, and rewarding to experience. It is a lifestyle change that will help you feel better, look better, and live better.

In this book, you will learn everything you need to know about the DASH diet and exercise program, including:

- The origins and principles of the DASH diet and exercise program
- The benefits of the DASH diet and exercise program for your health and well-being
- What to anticipate and how to use this book
- The foods to eat and avoid on the DASH diet
- How the DASH diet affects your blood pressure, weight, and overall health
- How to plan your meals and snacks on the DASH diet
- How to make healthy food choices on the DASH diet

- The best exercises to do on the DASH exercise program
- How the DASH exercise program boosts your metabolism, energy, and mood
- How to fit exercise into your busy schedule on the DASH exercise program
- How to find the right intensity and duration for your fitness level on the DASH exercise program
- How to track your progress and measure your results on the DASH diet and exercise program
- How to set realistic and achievable goals for the DASH diet and exercise program
- How to celebrate your successes on the DASH diet and exercise program
- The common challenges and pitfalls that you may encounter on the DASH diet and exercise program
- The strategies and solutions for overcoming them in the DASH diet and exercise program
- The tips and tricks for staying motivated and consistent on the DASH diet and exercise program
- How to make the DASH diet and exercise program a lifelong habit

- How to maintain the DASH diet and exercise program in different situations and seasons
- How to enjoy the DASH diet and exercise program and its lasting effects
- How to adapt the DASH diet and exercise program to your age, gender, health condition, and lifestyle
- The special considerations and precautions for different groups of people on the DASH diet and exercise program
- The success stories and testimonials of different people on the DASH diet and exercise program
- How to introduce the DASH diet and exercise program to children and adolescents
- How to tailor the DASH diet and exercise program to their specific needs and preferences
- How to support and encourage them on the DASH diet and exercise program
- How to deal with common issues and challenges for children and adolescents on the DASH diet and exercise program
- How to adjust the DASH diet and exercise program for seniors

- How to address the common health concerns and conditions for seniors on the DASH diet and exercise program
- How to help and motivate them on the DASH diet and exercise program
- How to cope with the changes and challenges for seniors on the DASH diet and exercise program
- The summary and review of the main points of the book
- The call to action and encouragement to start your DASH journey today

By the end of this book, you will have all the knowledge, skills, and tools you need to DASH your way to health and happiness. You will be able to follow the DASH diet and exercise program with confidence and ease, and you will enjoy the results for years to come. You will be able to transform your body, mind, and life with the power of DASH. Are you ready to DASH? Then let's get started!

The benefits of the DASH diet and exercise program for your health and well-being

The DASH diet and exercise program are not only effective for lowering your blood pressure but also for improving your overall health and well-being. By following the DASH diet and exercise program, you can enjoy the following benefits:

- **Weight loss and maintenance**: The DASH diet and exercise program can help you lose excess weight and keep it off, as it reduces your calorie intake and increases your energy expenditure. Losing weight can lower your blood pressure and reduce the risk of obesity-related diseases, such as diabetes, heart disease, and some cancers.
- **Cardiovascular health**: The DASH diet and exercise program can protect your heart and blood vessels, as it lowers your blood pressure, cholesterol, and triglycerides and prevents or reverses plaque buildup in your arteries. This can reduce the risk of heart attack, stroke, and heart failure and improve your heart function and quality of life.

- **Metabolic health:** The DASH diet and exercise program can improve your metabolism, as they enhance your insulin sensitivity and glucose tolerance and prevent or manage diabetes. This can prevent or delay the complications of diabetes, such as nerve damage, kidney damage, eye damage, and foot problems, and improve your blood sugar control and mood.

- **Kidney health**: The DASH diet and exercise program can preserve your kidney function, as it lowers your blood pressure and prevents or slows down the progression of kidney disease. This can prevent or delay the need for dialysis or transplantation and improve your fluid and electrolyte balance and waste removal.

- **Bone health:** The DASH diet and exercise program can strengthen your bones, as it provides adequate calcium, magnesium, vitamin D, and other nutrients and stimulates bone formation and density through weight-bearing exercise. This can prevent or treat osteoporosis and reduce the risk of fractures and falls.

- **Mental health:** The DASH diet and exercise program can boost your mood, as it provides antioxidants, omega-3 fatty acids, and other nutrients that support your brain health and function and releases endorphins and serotonin through physical activity. This can prevent or alleviate depression, anxiety, stress, and cognitive decline and improve your memory, attention, and learning.

What to anticipate and how to use this book

This book is your ultimate guide to the DASH diet and exercise program. It will give you all the information, advice, and resources you need to start and maintain your DASH journey. You can use this book in various ways, depending on your needs and preferences. You can read it from beginning to end, or you can jump to the chapters or sections that interest you the most. You can also use it as a reference book, and look up the answers to your questions or the reminders to your doubts. You can also use it as a workbook, and complete the exercises, quizzes, and charts that are provided throughout the book. You can also use it as a journal, and record your thoughts, feelings, and experiences on the DASH diet and exercise program. However you choose to use this book, you can expect to gain a lot, have fun, and see results. You can expect to improve your health and well-being, lower your blood pressure, lose weight, and enhance your metabolism and mood. You can expect to feel better, look better, and live better. You can expect to DASH your way to health and happiness.

CHAPTER 1

The DASH Diet: Eating for Optimal Health and Weight Loss

In this chapter, you will learn the basics of the DASH diet, which stands for Dietary Approaches to Stop Hypertension. The DASH diet is a healthy eating plan that can help you lower your blood pressure, lose weight, and improve your overall health. The DASH diet is based on scientific evidence and proven results, and it is recommended by many health organizations and experts. The DASH diet is not a restrictive or complicated diet. It is a balanced and flexible diet that emphasizes eating more fruits, vegetables, whole grains, low-fat dairy, lean protein, nuts, seeds, and legumes, and eating less salt, saturated fat, cholesterol, and sugar. The DASH diet also allows you to enjoy a variety of foods and flavors and to customize your diet according to your preferences and needs.

The DASH diet works by providing your body with the nutrients and antioxidants that it needs to function properly and to prevent or treat various health conditions. The DASH diet also helps you control your calorie intake and increase your satiety, which can help you lose weight and keep it off. By following the DASH diet, you can expect to see improvements in your blood pressure, weight, cholesterol, blood sugar, and more.

In this chapter, you will learn:

- The foods to eat and avoid on the DASH diet
- How the DASH diet affects your blood pressure, weight, and overall health
- How to plan your meals and snacks on the DASH diet
- How to make healthy food choices on the DASH diet

By the end of this chapter, you will have a clear understanding of the DASH diet and how to follow it. You will also have some practical tips and examples to help you get started and stay on track. You will be ready to DASH your way to optimal health and weight loss.

The foods to eat and avoid on the DASH diet

The DASH diet is based on eating more of the foods that are beneficial for your health and blood pressure and less of the foods that are harmful for them. The DASH diet does not require you to count calories or measure portions, but it does give you some general guidelines on how much of each food group you should eat per day. Here are the foods to eat and avoid on the DASH diet:

- **Fruits and vegetables**: Eat 4 to 5 servings of fruits and 4 to 5 servings of vegetables per day. Fruits and vegetables are rich in potassium, magnesium, fiber, and antioxidants, which help lower blood pressure and prevent oxidative damage. Choose fresh, frozen, or canned fruits and vegetables without added salt or sugar. Aim for a variety of colors and types, such as leafy greens, cruciferous vegetables, citrus fruits, berries, and melons.
- **Whole grains**: Eat 6 to 8 servings of whole grains per day. Whole grains are high in fiber, which helps lower cholesterol and blood sugar and keeps you full longer.

Choose whole wheat bread, pasta, and cereals; brown rice; oats; quinoa; barley; and other whole grains. Avoid refined grains, such as white bread, white rice, and pastries, which are low in fiber and nutrients and high in calories and sugar.

- **Low-fat dairy**: Eat 2 to 3 servings of low-fat dairy per day. Low-fat dairy is a good source of calcium, protein, and vitamin D, which help maintain bone health and muscle mass. Adopt the use of cottage cheese, yogurt, cheese, and milk that are low in fat or fat free.Avoid full-fat dairy, which is high in saturated fat and cholesterol and can boost the risk of heart disease and high blood pressure.

- **Lean protein**: Eat 6 or fewer servings of lean protein per day. Lean protein is essential for building and repairing tissues and for producing hormones and enzymes. Choose lean cuts of meat, poultry, and fish, such as chicken breast, turkey, salmon, tuna, and cod. Remove the skin and visible fat from meat and poultry, and bake, broil, grill, or roast them instead of frying. Limit your intake of red meat, such as beef, pork, and lamb, to no more than once or twice a week, as they are high in saturated fat and cholesterol. Avoid processed meats, such as bacon, ham, sausage, and hot dogs, which are high in sodium, nitrates, and preservatives and can increase blood pressure and cancer risk.

- **Nuts, seeds, and legumes**: Eat 4 to 5 servings of nuts, seeds, and legumes per week. Nuts, seeds, and legumes are rich in protein, fiber, healthy fats, and minerals, which help lower blood pressure, cholesterol, and inflammation. Choose almonds, walnuts, pistachios, sunflower seeds, pumpkin seeds, flaxseeds, chia seeds, beans, lentils, and soy products. Avoid salted, roasted, or candied nuts and seeds, which are high in sodium and sugar. Also, limit your intake of peanuts and peanut butter, which are high in calories and can cause allergic reactions in some people. Fats and oils: Eat 2 to 3 servings of fats and oils per day. Fats and oils are necessary for absorbing fat-soluble vitamins, such as A, D, E, and K, and for providing energy and cushioning for your organs. Choose healthy fats and oils, such as olive oil, canola oil, avocado, and nuts, which are high in monounsaturated and polyunsaturated fats and omega-3 fatty acids, which help lower blood pressure, cholesterol, and inflammation. Avoid unhealthy fats and oils, such as butter, margarine, lard, shortening, and coconut oil, which are high in saturated and trans fats and can raise blood pressure, cholesterol, and inflammation.

- **Sweets and added sugars**: Eat 5 or fewer servings of sweets and added sugars per week. Sweets and added sugars are high in calories and low in nutrients and can increase blood pressure, blood sugar, and weight. Choose natural sugars, such as fruits, honey, and maple syrup, which also provide some vitamins and minerals. Avoid artificial sugars, such as aspartame, sucralose, and saccharin, which can have negative effects on your health and appetite. Also, limit your intake of candies, chocolates, cakes, pies, cookies, ice cream, and other desserts, which are high in sugar, fat, and calories.

How the DASH diet affects your blood pressure, weight, and overall health

The DASH diet can have a positive impact on your blood pressure, weight, and overall health by providing your body with the nutrients and antioxidants that it needs to function properly and to prevent or treat various health conditions. Here are some of the ways that the DASH diet affects your health:

- **Blood pressure**: The DASH diet can lower your blood pressure by reducing the amount of sodium and increasing the amount of potassium, magnesium, and calcium in your diet. Sodium can raise blood pressure by causing your body to retain water and by constricting your blood vessels. Potassium, magnesium, and calcium can lower blood pressure by helping your body excrete excess sodium and by relaxing your blood vessels. By following the DASH diet, you can lower your systolic blood pressure (the top number) by 8 to 14 points and your diastolic blood pressure (the bottom number) by 4 to 9 points within two weeks.

- **Weight**: The DASH diet can help you lose weight and keep it off by reducing your calorie intake and increasing your satiety. The DASH diet is rich in fiber, which helps you feel full longer and prevents overeating. The DASH diet is also low in sugar, which helps you avoid blood sugar spikes, crashes, and cravings for sweets. The DASH diet also helps you burn more calories and fat by boosting your metabolism and providing lean protein, which helps you build and maintain muscle mass. By following the DASH diet, you can lose up to 10 pounds in 10 weeks and maintain a healthy weight for life.

- **Overall health**: The DASH diet can improve your overall health by preventing or managing chronic diseases such as cardiovascular disease, stroke, diabetes, and kidney disease. The DASH diet can also improve your blood cholesterol, insulin sensitivity, and antioxidant status, which are important indicators of your health. The DASH diet can also enhance your immune system, skin health, and mental health by providing vitamins, minerals, and phytochemicals that support your body's functions and protect it from damage and infection. By following the DASH diet, you can improve your quality of life and reduce your risk of premature death.

How to plan your meals and snacks on the DASH diet

Planning your meals and snacks on the DASH diet can help you stick to your eating plan, avoid temptation, and save time and money. Here are some tips on how to plan your meals and snacks on the DASH diet:

- **Use the DASH diet food pyramid as a guide**. The DASH diet food pyramid shows you how many servings of each food group you should eat per day, and what a serving size looks like. You can use the pyramid to plan your meals and snacks, and to balance your intake of different nutrients.

- **Plan ahead and make a list.** Before you go grocery shopping, plan your meals and snacks for the week, and make a list of the ingredients you need. This will help you avoid buying unnecessary or unhealthy items, and save you time and money.

- Prepare your meals and snacks in advance. If you have some free time, you can prepare your meals and snacks in advance, and store them in the fridge or freezer. This will make it easier for you to eat healthy and avoid skipping meals or snacking on junk food. You can also use batch cooking, freezer meals, or meal prep containers to make your meals and snacks ahead of time.

- Prepare meals and snacks for the office or classroom. If you are going to work or school, you can pack your meals and snacks in a cooler bag, a lunch box, or a thermos. This will help you avoid eating out or vending machines, and save you money and calories. You can also pack some extra servings of fruits, vegetables, nuts, seeds, and low-fat dairy, in case you get hungry between meals

How to make healthy food choices on the DASH diet

Making healthy food choices on the DASH diet can help you optimize your nutrition, flavor, and satisfaction. Here are some tips on how to make healthy food choices on the DASH diet:

- **Choose whole foods over processed foods.** Whole foods are foods that are in their natural or minimally processed state, such as fruits, vegetables, whole grains, nuts, seeds, and legumes. Processed foods are foods that have been altered or modified by adding or removing ingredients, such as salt, sugar, fat, preservatives, or artificial colors and flavors. Whole foods are more nutritious, filling, and tasty than processed foods, and they contain less sodium, sugar, fat, and calories. For example, choose an apple over apple juice, brown rice over white rice, or oatmeal over cereal.

- **Choose low-sodium or sodium-free options.** Sodium can cause blood pressure to rise, as well as increasing the risk of heart disease and stroke. The DASH diet recommends limiting your sodium intake to no more than 2,300 mg per day, or 1,500 mg if you have high blood pressure or are at risk of developing it. To reduce your sodium intake, choose fresh, frozen, or canned foods without added salt, rinse canned foods to remove excess salt, avoid or limit salty foods such as chips, pretzels, pickles, soy sauce, and cheese, use herbs, spices, lemon juice, vinegar, or salt-free seasoning blends to flavor your food, and read nutrition labels and choose products with less than 140 mg of sodium per serving.

- Choose low-fat or fat-free dairy products. Dairy products are a good source of calcium, protein, and vitamin D, which are important for your bone health and muscle mass. However, dairy products can also be high in saturated fat and cholesterol, which can raise your blood pressure and increase your risk of heart disease. The DASH diet recommends choosing low-fat or fat-free dairy products,

CHAPTER 2
The DASH Exercise Program: Moving for Enhanced Metabolism and Mood

In this chapter, you will learn the basics of the DASH exercise program, which is a complementary and integral part of the DASH diet and lifestyle. The DASH exercise program is a moderate-intensity physical activity program that can help you lower your blood pressure, lose weight, and improve your metabolism and mood. The DASH exercise program is based on scientific evidence and proven results, and it is recommended by many health organizations and experts.

The DASH exercise program is not a strenuous or complicated exercise program. It is a simple and flexible exercise program that emphasizes doing more of the activities that you enjoy and less of the activities that you dread. The DASH exercise program also allows you to adjust the type, frequency, intensity, and duration of your exercise according to your preferences and needs.

The DASH exercise program works by providing your body with the stimulation and challenge that it needs to function optimally and to adapt to stress. The DASH exercise program also helps you burn more calories and fat, build and tone your muscles, strengthen your heart and lungs, and boost your mood and energy. By following the DASH exercise program, you can expect to see improvements in your blood pressure, weight, cholesterol, blood sugar, and more.

By the end of this chapter, you will have a clear understanding of the DASH exercise program and how to follow it. You will also have some practical tips and examples to help you get started and stay on track. You will be ready to DASH your way to enhanced metabolism and mood.

The best exercises to do on the DASH exercise program

The DASH exercise program does not prescribe a specific type of exercise, but rather a general level of intensity and duration. The best exercises to do on the DASH exercise program are the ones that you enjoy, that suit your fitness level, and that challenge your heart and muscles. However, some exercises are more beneficial than others for lowering your blood pressure, losing weight, and improving your metabolism and mood. Here are some examples of the best exercises to do on the DASH exercise program:

- **Aerobic exercises:** These are exercises that increase your heart rate and breathing and use large muscle groups, such as your legs, arms, and chest. Aerobic exercises can lower your blood pressure, burn calories and fat, and boost your mood and energy. Some examples of aerobic exercises are brisk walking, jogging, cycling, swimming, dancing, or skipping rope. At least 150 minutes of moderate-intensity aerobic activity, 75 minutes of vigorous-intensity aerobic exercise, or a mix of the two, should be your weekly goal.
- **Strength training exercises:** These are exercises that use resistance, such as weights, bands, or your own body weight, to work your muscles. Strength training exercises can increase your metabolism, muscle mass, and bone density and improve your posture and

balance. Some examples of strength training exercises are squats, lunges, push-ups, pull-ups, planks, or bicep curls. You should aim for at least two sessions of strength training per week, targeting all major muscle groups.

- **Flexibility and balance exercises:** These are exercises that improve your range of motion, prevent injuries, reduce stress, and enhance your coordination and stability. Flexibility and balance exercises can also lower your blood pressure by relaxing your blood vessels and improving your blood flow. Some examples of flexibility and balance exercises are stretching, yoga, tai chi, or pilates. You should aim for at least two sessions of flexibility and balance exercises per week, or more often if you can.

How the DASH exercise program boosts your metabolism, energy, and mood

The DASH exercise program can boost your metabolism, energy, and mood by stimulating your body's physiological and psychological processes. Here are some of the ways that the DASH exercise program boosts your health and well-being:

- **Metabolism:** The DASH exercise program can increase your metabolic rate, which is the amount of calories and fat that your body burns at rest and during activity. By doing aerobic exercises, you can increase your oxygen consumption and calorie expenditure, and by doing strength training exercises, you can increase your muscle mass and calorie burning. By increasing your metabolism, you can lose weight, prevent weight gain, and improve your blood sugar control and insulin sensitivity.
- **Energy:** The DASH exercise program can increase your energy levels, which is the amount of physical and mental stamina that you have throughout the day. By doing aerobic exercises, you can improve your

cardiovascular fitness and endurance, and by doing strength training exercises, you can improve your muscular strength and power. By increasing your energy levels, you can perform better at work, school, or daily activities and reduce your fatigue and tiredness.

- **Mood:** The DASH exercise program can improve your mood, which is the state of your emotions and feelings. By doing aerobic exercises, you can release endorphins and serotonin, which are natural chemicals that make you feel happy and relaxed, and by doing strength training exercises, you can release dopamine and norepinephrine, which are natural chemicals that make you feel alert and motivated. By improving your mood, you can reduce your stress, anxiety, and depression and enhance your self-esteem and confidence.

How to fit exercise into your busy schedule with the DASH exercise program

One of the common challenges that people face when trying to adopt a healthier lifestyle is finding time to exercise. You may have a hectic work schedule, family obligations, or other commitments that make it hard to squeeze in a workout. However, there are some simple and effective ways to fit exercise into your busy schedule on the DASH exercise program. Here are some tips to help you:

- **Plan ahead.** At the beginning of each week, look at your calendar and identify the gaps in your schedule where you can fit in some exercise. Block out those times and treat them as appointments that you can't miss. To help you stay on task, you may also program reminders on your computer or phone.

- **Be flexible**. Sometimes, things may not go according to plan, and you may have to skip or reschedule your workout. Don't let that discourage you or make you give up. Instead, look for another opportunity to exercise later in the day or week. You can also split your workout into shorter sessions throughout the day, such as 10 minutes in the morning, 10 minutes at lunch, and 10 minutes in the evening.

- **Make it convenient.** Choose an exercise that you enjoy and that is easy to do anywhere, such as walking, jogging, cycling, or skipping. You can also invest in some portable equipment, such as resistance bands, dumbbells, or a jump rope, that you can use at home, at work, or while traveling. Alternatively, you can use online videos, apps, or podcasts that guide you through different workouts that you can do with minimal or no equipment.

- **Use your commute**. If you drive to work, park your car farther away from your office and walk the rest of the way. If you take public transportation, get off a stop earlier and walk the remaining distance. If you live close enough to your workplace, consider biking or walking instead of driving or taking the bus. These are simple ways to add some extra physical activity to your daily routine.

- **Take advantage of your breaks.** Whether you work in an office or from home, you can use your breaks to get some exercise. For example, you can walk around the block, climb the stairs, do some stretches, or perform some bodyweight exercises, such as squats, lunges, push-ups, or planks. You can also join a colleague or a friend for a quick walk or a workout session during your break. This will not only help you burn some calories but also boost your mood and productivity.

- **Make it fun**. Workouts don't have to be monotonous or boring. You can make it more enjoyable and rewarding by adding some variety, challenge, and fun to your routine. For example, you can try a new activity, such as dancing, yoga, or martial arts, that interests you. You can also join a group, a class, or a club that offers social support and accountability. You can also set some goals, track your progress, and reward yourself for your achievements.

How to make healthy food choices on the DASH diet

One of the main features of the DASH diet is that it emphasizes healthy food choices that are low in salt, saturated fat, and added sugar and high in potassium, calcium, magnesium, fiber, and protein. These nutrients can help lower your blood pressure, cholesterol, and weight, and improve your overall health and well-being. However, making healthy food choices on the DASH diet may not always be easy or obvious, especially if you are used to eating processed, fast, or convenience foods. Here are some tips to help you make healthy food choices on the DASH diet:

1. Choose fresh fruits and vegetables (or frozen with no added salt), whole grains, beans and legumes, fish, lean meats, and nuts (with no added salt). These foods are rich in the minerals and fiber that the DASH diet recommends and can also provide antioxidants, phytochemicals, and other beneficial compounds that can protect your health. You should aim for at least four or five servings of fruits and vegetables daily

and six to eight servings of whole grains per day.

2. Avoid or limit foods that are high in salt, saturated fat, and added sugar, such as processed meats, cheese, butter, pastries, candies, sodas, and chips. These foods can increase your blood pressure, cholesterol, and weight and contribute to inflammation, oxidative stress, and other health problems. You should limit your salt intake to no more than 2,300 mg per day, or 1,500 mg per day if you have high blood pressure or are at risk of developing it. You should also limit your saturated fat intake to less than 10% of your total calories per day and your added sugar intake to less than 10% of your total calories per day.

3. Read nutrition labels and ingredient lists carefully. Nutrition labels can help you compare different products and choose the ones that are lower in salt, saturated fat, and added sugar and higher in potassium, calcium, magnesium, fiber, and protein. Ingredient lists can help you identify the sources and types of salt, fat, and sugar in the product and avoid any additives,

preservatives, or artificial flavors or colors that you may want to avoid. You should also pay attention to the serving size and the number of servings per container, as they may differ from what you normally eat.

4. Cook your own meals and snacks as much as possible. Cooking your own food can give you more control over the ingredients, portions, and flavors of your meals and snacks. You can use fresh, whole, and natural ingredients and avoid or limit salt, saturated fat, and added sugar. You can also use herbs, spices, vinegar, lemon juice, or other seasonings to enhance the taste and aroma of your food without adding extra salt or calories. You can also prepare your food in healthy ways, such as steaming, baking, broiling, or grilling, instead of frying or deep-frying.

5. Plan ahead and be prepared. Planning your meals and snacks ahead of time can help you stick to the DASH diet and avoid temptations or cravings. You can make a weekly menu, a shopping list, and a budget, and stock up on healthy foods and ingredients. You can also cook in bulk and freeze or refrigerate the

leftovers for later use. You can also pack your own lunch and snacks and bring them to work, school, or wherever you go. This way, you can avoid eating out or ordering takeout, which may not offer healthy options or portions.

CHAPTER 3

Tracking Your Progress and Measuring Your Results: Setting goals and celebrating successes

One of the most important aspects of following the DASH diet and exercise program is tracking your progress and measuring your results. This can help you stay motivated, focused, and accountable, as well as evaluate your strengths and weaknesses and adjust your plan accordingly. Tracking your progress and measuring your results can also help you set realistic and achievable goals and celebrate your successes along the way. This chapter will teach you how to track your progress on the DASH diet and exercise program using various tools and methods, such as journals, apps, trackers, scales, and tests, measure your results on the DASH diet and exercise program using various indicators and metrics, such as blood pressure, weight, body fat, waist circumference, and fitness level, set realistic and achievable goals on the DASH diet and exercise program using the SMART (Specific, Measurable, Attainable, Relevant, and Time-bound) framework, celebrate your successes on the DASH diet and exercise program using various strategies and rewards, such as acknowledging your efforts, sharing your achievements, treating yourself, and reflecting on your journey.

By the end of this chapter, you will have a clear and comprehensive understanding of how to track your progress and measure your results on the DASH diet and exercise program and how to use this information to set goals and celebrate successes. This will help you make the most of the DASH diet and exercise program and enjoy its benefits for your health and happiness.

How to track your progress on the DASH diet and exercise program

Tracking your progress on the DASH diet and exercise program can help you stay motivated, focused, and accountable. It can also help you evaluate your strengths and weaknesses and adjust your plan accordingly. There are various tools and methods that you can use to track your progress, such as:

- **Journals**. You can use a journal to record your daily food intake, physical activity, blood pressure, weight, and other relevant information. Another option is to record your emotions, ideas, difficulties, and accomplishments. A journal can help you monitor your habits, identify patterns, and reflect on your journey.

- **Trackers**. You can use a tracker, such as a pedometer, a smartwatch, or a wearable device, to measure your physical activity, such as your steps, distance, speed, calories, and heart rate. A tracker can help you set and achieve your activity goals and motivate you to move more.

- **Scales**. You can use a scale, such as a digital or smart scale, to measure your weight, body fat, muscle mass, and other body composition indicators. A scale can help you track your weight loss or gain and assess your health and fitness level.

- **Tests.** You can use a test, such as a blood pressure test, a blood glucose test, a cholesterol test, or a fitness test, to measure your health and fitness parameters, such as your blood pressure, blood sugar, cholesterol, or aerobic capacity. A test can help you track your health and fitness improvements and detect any problems or risks.

These are some of the tools and methods that you can use to track your progress on the DASH diet and exercise program. You can choose the ones that suit your needs, preferences, and budget, and use them regularly and consistently. By tracking your progress, you can see how far you have come and how much further you can go.

How to measure your results on the DASH diet and exercise program

Measuring your results on the DASH diet and exercise program can help you evaluate your health and fitness improvements and detect any problems or risks. It can also help you set and adjust your goals and celebrate your achievements. There are various indicators and metrics that you can use to measure your results, such as:

-**Blood pressure**. Blood pressure is one of the main indicators of your cardiovascular health and the primary target of the DASH diet and exercise program. You can measure your blood pressure using a home monitor, a pharmacy machine, or a doctor's office device. You should measure your blood pressure at the same time of the day, preferably in the morning, and follow the instructions carefully. You should aim for a blood pressure below 120/80 mmHg, which is considered normal for adults. If your blood pressure is above 140/90 mmHg, you have high blood pressure, and you may need to consult your doctor for further treatment.

- **Weight**. Weight is another indicator of your health and fitness, and it is a secondary target of the DASH diet and exercise program. You can measure your weight using a digital or smart scale, preferably in the morning, before eating or drinking, and wearing minimal clothing. You should weigh yourself once a week and record your weight in a journal or an app. You should aim for a healthy weight range based on your height, age, and gender. A common way to determine your healthy weight range is to calculate your body mass index (BMI), which is your weight in kilograms divided by your height in meters squared. A normal BMI range for adults is between 18.5 and 24.9. If your BMI is below 18.5, you are underweight, and if your BMI is above 25, you are overweight or obese.

Body fat. Body fat is a more accurate indicator of your health and fitness than weight, as it reflects the amount of fat tissue in your body, which can affect your metabolism, hormones, and inflammation. You can measure your body fat using a body fat analyzer, a skinfold caliper, or a bioelectrical impedance device. You should measure your body fat at the same time of the day, preferably in the morning, and follow the instructions carefully. You should aim for a healthy body fat percentage based on your age and gender. A general guideline for healthy body fat percentage for adults is between 10% and 20% for men and between 18% and 28% for women.

waist circumference. Waist circumference is another indicator of your health and fitness, as it reflects the amount of visceral fat in your abdomen, which can increase your risk of diabetes, heart disease, and stroke. You can measure your waist circumference using a tape measure, preferably in the morning, and follow the instructions carefully. You should measure your waist circumference at the level of your navel and breathe normally. You should aim for a healthy waist circumference based on your gender. A general guideline for healthy waist circumference for adults is less than 40 inches (102 cm) for men and less than 35 inches (88 cm) for women.

fitness level. Fitness level is another indicator of your health and fitness, as it reflects your aerobic and anaerobic capacity, strength, endurance, and flexibility. You can measure your fitness level using various tests, such as a step test, a push-up test, a sit-up test, or a sit-and-reach test. You should perform these tests at the same time of the day, preferably in the morning, and follow the instructions carefully. You should compare your results with the normative data based on your age and gender and aim for a good or excellent fitness level.

How to celebrate your successes on the DASH diet and exercise program

Celebrating your successes on the DASH diet and exercise program can help you stay motivated, focused, and accountable. It can also help you acknowledge your efforts and achievements and reward yourself for your hard work. However, celebrating your successes does not mean that you have to undo your progress or compromise your goals. Therefore, it is important to use smart and effective celebration strategies, such as:

-**Acknowledge your efforts.** Recognize and appreciate the positive changes that you have made to your diet and exercise habits, and how they have improved your health and well-being. You can use a journal, an app, a tracker, or a test to record and review your progress and results and see how far you have come and how much further you can go.

Share your achievements. Tell your family, friends, co-workers, or online community about your successes, and ask for their support and feedback. You can also join a group, a class, or a club that follows the DASH diet and exercise program and share your experiences, challenges, and tips with other like-minded people.

-Treat yourself. Reward yourself with something that makes you happy and satisfied but does not sabotage your diet and exercise plan. For example, you can buy yourself a new outfit, book, or gadget, or treat yourself to a massage, a movie, or a concert. You can also indulge in a small portion of your favorite food or drink, as long as you balance it with healthy choices and moderation.

-Reflect on your journey. Think about the reasons why you started the DASH diet and exercise program and how it has changed your life for the better. Think about the challenges that you have overcome and the lessons that you have learned. Think about the goals that you have achieved and the ones that you still want to pursue. Think about the benefits that you have gained and the ones that you still want to enjoy.

-Recognize your efforts. Give yourself credit and praise for the positive changes that you have made to your diet and exercise habits and how they have improved your health and well-being. You can use a journal, an app, a tracker, or a test to record and review your progress and results and see how far you have come and how much further you can go.

-Tell about your achievements. Share your successes with your family, friends, co-workers, or online community, and ask for their support and feedback. You can also join a group, a class, or a club that follows the DASH diet and exercise program and share your experiences, challenges, and tips with other like-minded people. You can also inspire and motivate others by sharing your story and testimonial on the web.

-Reward yourself. Treat yourself to something that makes you happy and satisfied but does not sabotage your diet and exercise plan. For example, you can buy yourself a new outfit, book, or gadget, or treat yourself to a massage, a movie, or a concert. You can also indulge in a small portion of your favorite food or drink, as long as you balance it with healthy choices and moderation.

-Reflect on your journey. Think about the reasons why you started the DASH diet and exercise program and how it has changed your life for the better. Think about the challenges that you have overcome and the lessons that you have learned.

Think about the goals that you have achieved and the ones that you still want to pursue. Think about the benefits that you have gained and the ones that you still want to enjoy. These are some of the ways to celebrate your successes on the DASH diet and exercise program. By celebrating your successes, you can reinforce your positive behavior, boost your self-esteem, and enhance your happiness.

These are some of the ways to celebrate your successes on the DASH diet and exercise program. By celebrating your successes, you can reinforce your positive behavior, boost your self-esteem, and enhance your happiness.

How to set realistic and achievable goals on the DASH diet and exercise program

Setting realistic and achievable goals on the DASH diet and exercise program can help you stay motivated, focused, and accountable. It can also help you measure your progress and results and celebrate your successes. However, setting goals that are too vague, unrealistic, or unattainable can lead to frustration, disappointment, and failure. Therefore, it is important to use a smart and effective goal-setting strategy, such as the SMART goal framework. Here is how to apply the SMART framework to your goals on the DASH diet and exercise program:

-**Specific:** Your goals should be clear and defined, not vague or general. Speak like this instead of merely saying, "I want to eat healthier": "I want to eat four servings of fruits and vegetables every day."

-**Measurable:** Rather than being arbitrary or subjective, your objectives should be measurable and observable. For example, instead of saying "I want to exercise more," say "I want to walk for 30 minutes five times a week.".

-**Attainable:** Your goals should be realistic and achievable, not impossible or out of reach. For instance, say, "I want to lose 10 pounds in 3 months" rather than "I want to lose 50 pounds in a month.".

-**Relevant:** Your goals should be meaningful and aligned with your values, interests, and needs, not irrelevant or unrelated. For instance, as opposed to expressing "I want to lower my blood pressure because my doctor told me to," declare "I want to lower my blood pressure because I want to prevent heart disease and stroke.".

-**Time-bound:** Your goals should have a specific deadline or timeframe, not be indefinite or open-ended.

For example, instead of saying "I want to lower my cholesterol," say "I want to lower my cholesterol by 20 points by December 31st.". These are some of the ways to set realistic and achievable goals for the DASH diet and exercise program using the SMART framework. By setting SMART goals, you can create a clear and concrete plan of action and monitor and achieve your desired outcomes. You can also review and revise your goals as needed, and adjust your plan accordingly. By setting SMART goals, you can make the most of the DASH diet and exercise program and improve your health and happiness.

CHAPTER 4

Overcoming Common Challenges and Pitfalls: Dealing with Cravings, Plateaus, Boredom, and More

One of the most challenging aspects of following the DASH diet and exercise program is overcoming the common challenges and pitfalls that you may encounter along the way. These challenges and pitfalls can include cravings, plateaus, boredom, a lack of time, a lack of support, and more. These challenges and pitfalls can affect your motivation, consistency, and results, and make you feel like giving up. However, there are some effective strategies and solutions that can help you overcome these challenges and pitfalls and stay on track with the DASH diet and exercise program. This chapter will teach you how to:

- Deal with cravings. Cravings are the intense urges or desires to eat or drink something that is not part of your diet plan, such as sweets, salty snacks, or alcohol. Cravings can be triggered by various factors, such as stress, emotions, hormones, habits, or environmental cues. Cravings can make you lose control, overeat, and sabotage your diet and health goals.

- Break through plateaus. Plateaus are the periods of time when your progress and results seem to stall or slow down despite following your diet and exercise plan. Plateaus can be caused by various factors, such as metabolic adaptation, muscle loss, water retention, or measurement errors. Plateaus can make you feel frustrated and discouraged and doubt your efforts and abilities.

- Avoid boredom. Boredom is the feeling of being tired or uninterested in your diet and exercise routine due to a lack of variety, challenge, or fun. Boredom can make you lose interest and enthusiasm and seek other sources of stimulation or satisfaction, such as unhealthy foods or activities.

- Manage your time. Time is the amount of available or free time that you have to devote to your diet and exercise plan, which can be limited by various factors, such as work, family, or other commitments. Time can make you feel overwhelmed and stressed, and you can neglect your diet and exercise priorities.

- Seek support. Support is the amount and quality of help, encouragement, or feedback that you receive from others, such as your family, friends, co-workers, or online community, regarding your diet and exercise plan. Support can make you feel more confident and accountable, and less isolated and lonely.

These are some of the common challenges and pitfalls that you may encounter on the DASH diet and exercise program and how to overcome them. By overcoming these challenges and pitfalls, you can maintain your motivation and consistency and achieve your desired outcomes. You can also enjoy the DASH diet and exercise program and its benefits for your health and happiness.

The strategies and solutions for overcoming the common challenges and pitfalls of the DASH diet and exercise program

The DASH diet and exercise program can help you lower your blood pressure and improve your health, but they may also pose some challenges and pitfalls that can hinder your success. However, you can overcome them by applying some strategies and solutions that are based on scientific evidence and practical experience. Some of them are:

- **Cravings:** To overcome cravings, you should first identify the triggers and patterns that cause them, such as stress, boredom, hunger, or emotions. Then, you should find healthy ways to cope with them, such as drinking water, chewing gum, meditating, or distracting yourself with a hobby. You should also plan ahead and have healthy snacks ready, such as fruits, nuts, or granola bars, to satisfy your hunger and prevent overeating. You should also avoid skipping meals, as this can make you more prone to cravings and binge eating. Finally, you should reward yourself for resisting cravings, such as by giving yourself a compliment, a sticker, or a small treat.

- **Plateaus:** To overcome plateaus, you should first reassess your goals and progress and make sure that you are measuring them accurately and realistically. You should use multiple indicators, such as weight, blood pressure, waist circumference, body fat percentage, and fitness level, to track your improvement. You should also celebrate your achievements, no matter how small, and remind yourself of the benefits of the DASH diet and exercise program. Then, you should make some adjustments to your diet and exercise plan, such as by reducing your calorie intake, increasing your physical activity, changing the type, intensity, frequency, or duration of your exercises, or adding some resistance training or high-intensity interval training. You should also monitor your food intake and physical activity and keep a journal or use an app to record them. This can help you identify areas that need improvement and keep you accountable and motivated.

- **Boredom:** To overcome boredom, you should try to make your diet and exercise program more fun and enjoyable. You should experiment with different recipes, spices, herbs, and flavors to make your meals more exciting and delicious. You can also try new foods, such as ethnic cuisines, exotic fruits, or superfoods, to add some variety and novelty to your diet. You should also try new activities, such as swimming, dancing, cycling, or yoga, to keep your body and mind engaged and stimulated. You can also join a class, a club, or a team to meet new people, learn new skills, and have some social support and interaction. You can also set some challenges, such as running a 5K, lifting a certain weight, or cooking a new dish, to keep yourself challenged and motivated.

- **Social pressure:** To overcome social pressure, you should try to communicate with your family, friends, or coworkers and explain to them why you are following the DASH diet and exercise program and how it benefits your health and well-being. You should also ask them to respect your choices and to support you by joining you in your healthy habits, or at least not interfere with them. You should also seek out people who share your goals and values, such as online communities, support groups, or fitness buddies, who can offer you encouragement, advice, and accountability. You should also be confident and assertive and stand up for yourself and your decisions. You should also be flexible and adaptable and find ways to enjoy the DASH diet and exercise program in different situations and seasons, such as by bringing your own food, ordering wisely, or modifying your exercises.

The tips and tricks for staying motivated and consistent on the DASH diet and exercise program

The DASH diet and exercise program can help you lower your blood pressure and improve your health, but it may also require some commitment and discipline from you. To stay motivated and consistent on the DASH diet and exercise program, you should follow some tips and tricks that are based on psychological principles and behavioral science. Some of them are:

- **Set SMART goals:** SMART, as an abbreviation, stands for Specific, Measurable, Achievable, Relevant, and Time-bound. You should set SMART goals for your DASH diet and exercise program, such as "I will lose 10 pounds in 3 months by following the DASH diet and exercising for 30 minutes five times a week." SMART goals can assist you in setting clear expectations, monitoring your development, and acknowledging your successes.
- **Use positive affirmations:** Positive affirmations are statements that you repeat to

yourself to boost your confidence and motivation, such as "I am strong and healthy," "I can do this," or "I deserve to be happy." Positive affirmations can help you overcome negative thoughts, emotions, and beliefs and reinforce your self-esteem and self-efficacy.

- **Visualize your success:** Visualization is a technique that involves imagining yourself achieving your desired outcome, such as lowering your blood pressure, fitting into your favorite clothes, or feeling energetic and vibrant. Visualization can help you create a mental image of your goal and activate the same brain regions that are involved in the actual performance. This can enhance your motivation, focus, and performance.

- **Find your why:** Your why is the reason or purpose behind your DASH diet and exercise program, such as improving your health, preventing diseases, or living longer. Your why can help you connect your DASH diet and exercise program to your values, passions, and aspirations and inspire you to keep going when you face challenges or temptations.

- **Reward yourself:** Rewards are incentives that you give yourself for achieving your goals or completing your tasks, such as buying yourself a new book, watching a movie, or getting a massage. Rewards can help you reinforce your positive behaviors, increase your satisfaction, and maintain your motivation.

How to enjoy the DASH diet and exercise program and its lasting effects

The DASH diet and exercise program is not only a way to lower your blood pressure and improve your health, but also a way to enhance your quality of life and happiness. You can enjoy the DASH diet and exercise program and its lasting effects by following some tips and tricks that are based on positive psychology and wellness research. Some of them are:

- **Focus on the process, not the outcome:** Instead of obsessing over the numbers on the scale or the blood pressure monitor, you should focus on the process of following the DASH diet and exercise program, and the positive changes that it brings to your body and mind. You should appreciate the journey, and the learning and growth that it entails. You should also celebrate every step and milestone that you achieve, and acknowledge your efforts and achievements.

- **Be mindful and present:** You should be mindful and present when you eat and exercise, and pay attention to your sensations, emotions, and thoughts. You should savor the flavors, textures, and aromas of your food, and enjoy the movement, energy, and strength of your body. You should also be aware of your hunger and fullness cues, and listen to your body's needs and preferences. You should also be grateful for the food that nourishes you, and the exercise that invigorates you.

- **Be positive and optimistic:** You should be positive and optimistic about the DASH diet and exercise program, and its effects on your health and well-being. You should have a positive attitude and outlook, and believe in your ability and potential. You should also avoid negative self-talk, and replace it with positive affirmations. You should also look for the bright side and the silver lining in every situation, and see challenges as opportunities, not obstacles.

- **Be social and supportive:** You should be social and supportive when you follow the DASH diet and exercise program, and share your experiences and goals with others. You should seek out people who share your values and aspirations, such as online communities, support groups, or fitness buddies, who can offer you encouragement, advice, and accountability. You should also involve your family, friends, or coworkers, and invite them to join you in your healthy habits, or at least support you in your choices. You should also be supportive of others, and offer them help, feedback, and recognition.

How to maintain the DASH diet and exercise program in different situations and seasons

The DASH diet and exercise program is a flexible and adaptable way to lower your blood pressure and improve your health, but it may also require some adjustments and modifications depending on the situation and season that you are in. You can maintain the DASH diet and exercise program in different situations and seasons by following some tips and tricks that are based on common sense and practical experience. Some of them are:

- **Traveling:** When you are traveling, you may face some challenges in following the DASH diet and exercise program, such as limited food choices, unfamiliar cuisines, or disrupted routines. To cope with these challenges, you should plan ahead and research the food options and availability at your destination, and pack some healthy snacks and water for the journey. You should also be flexible and adventurous, and try some local dishes that are low in salt, fat, and sugar, and high in fruits, vegetables, and whole grains. You should also be mindful and moderate, and avoid overeating or indulging in unhealthy foods, and balance them with some physical activity. You should also maintain your exercise routine as much as possible, and look for opportunities to move your body, such as walking, hiking, swimming, or sightseeing.
- **Holidays:** When you are celebrating holidays, you may face some temptations in following the DASH diet and exercise

program, such as festive foods, drinks, or desserts, or social gatherings, parties, or events. To resist these temptations, you should set some boundaries and limits, and decide in advance what and how much you will eat and drink, and stick to your plan. You should also be selective and sensible, and choose the foods and drinks that you enjoy the most, and savor them slowly and mindfully. You should also be active and sociable, and focus on the people and the occasion, rather than the food and the drink. You should also keep up your exercise routine as much as possible, and make it fun and festive, such as by playing some games, dancing, or decorating.

- **Seasons:** When you are experiencing different seasons, you may face some variations in following the DASH diet and exercise program, such as seasonal foods, weather, or mood. To adapt to these variations, you should embrace and enjoy the diversity and richness of each season, and use it to your advantage. You should eat seasonally and locally, and take advantage of the fresh and abundant fruits, vegetables, and herbs that each season offers. You should also exercise seasonally and appropriately, and adjust your activities and clothing to the weather and the temperature. You should also manage your mood and energy, and cope with any seasonal affective disorder or fatigue that you may experience, by getting enough sunlight, sleep, and relaxation.

CHAPTER 5

Making the DASH Diet and Exercise Program a Lifelong Habit: Tips and Tricks for Staying Motivated and Consistent

You have learned about the benefits of the DASH diet and exercise program and how to overcome the common challenges and pitfalls that you may encounter along the way. You have also learned how to enjoy the DASH diet and exercise program, its lasting effects, and how to maintain it in different situations and seasons. But how do you make the DASH diet and exercise program a lifelong habit and not just a temporary fix? How do you ensure that you stick to it for the long term and do not fall back into your old habits?

In this chapter, you will discover the secrets of habit formation and behavior change and how to apply them to the DASH diet and exercise program. You will learn how to create and sustain healthy habits that are aligned with your goals and values, and how to break and replace unhealthy habits that are holding you back. You will also learn how to use various tools and techniques, such as cues, rewards, routines, reminders, feedback, and support, to reinforce your habits and make them automatic and effortless. By the end of this chapter, you will have the skills and knowledge to make the DASH diet and exercise program a lifelong habit and enjoy its benefits for the rest of your life.

How to make the DASH diet and exercise program a lifelong habit

The DASH diet and exercise program are not just a temporary fix for your blood pressure or weight. It is a lifestyle change that can improve your overall health, well-being, and quality of life. But how do you make it a lifelong habit? Here are some tips and tricks to help you stay motivated and consistent on the DASH diet and exercise program.

- **Set realistic and specific goals.** Having a clear and attainable goal can help you focus on your progress and achievements. For example, instead of saying "I want to lower my blood pressure," you can say "I want to lower my blood pressure by 10 points in 3 months." This way, you can measure your success and adjust your plan accordingly.

- **Find physical activities that you enjoy.** Exercise is an essential part of the DASH diet and exercise program, as it can lower your blood pressure, improve your cardiovascular health, and burn calories. But exercise does not have to be boring or tedious. You can find physical activities that suit your preferences, abilities, and schedule. For example, you can try walking, jogging, cycling, swimming, dancing, yoga, pilates, or any other sport or hobby that gets you moving. You can also vary your routine, challenge yourself, and have fun with your exercise.

- **Create a supportive environment.** Surrounding yourself with people and things that encourage and inspire you can help you stay on track with the DASH diet and exercise program. You can seek support from your family, friends, co-workers, or online community, who can offer you advice, feedback, accountability, and companionship. You can also create a positive and healthy environment at home, work, and other places where you can access the resources and tools that you need for the DASH diet and exercise program, such as cookbooks, recipes, equipment, apps, etc.

- **Find a buddy or a group.** Having a buddy or a group that shares your goals and interests can make the DASH diet and exercise program more enjoyable and effective. You can find a buddy or a group that can join you for your meals, snacks, and physical activities and motivate you to stick to the DASH diet and exercise program. You can also exchange tips, ideas, experiences, and stories with your buddy or group and learn from each other. You can find a buddy or a group online, offline, or both, depending on your preference and availability.

- **Use reminders and rewards.** Reminding yourself of your reasons and benefits for following the DASH diet and exercise program can help you stay focused and motivated. You can use reminders such as notes, posters, pictures, quotes, or affirmations that can remind you of your goals, values, and achievements. You can also use rewards such as stickers, badges, points, or prizes that can reward you for your efforts, actions, and outcomes. You can use reminders and rewards that are meaningful and appealing to you and place them where you can see them often.

How to maintain the DASH diet and exercise program in different situations and seasons

The DASH diet and exercise program can be adapted to different situations and seasons, so you don't have to worry about losing your momentum or missing out on the benefits. Here are some tips and tricks to help you maintain the DASH diet and exercise program in various scenarios:

- **When you are traveling.** Traveling can be a challenge for the DASH diet and exercise program, as you may face unfamiliar foods, limited options, and disrupted routines. But you can still follow the DASH diet and exercise program with some planning and preparation. You can pack some healthy snacks, such as fruits, nuts, granola bars, or crackers, to keep you satisfied on the road or in the air. You can also research the local cuisine and culture and look for dishes that are low in sodium, saturated fat, and added sugars and high in potassium, calcium, magnesium, fiber, and protein. You can also ask for modifications, such as less salt, oil, or sauce, or more vegetables, when ordering your food. For exercise, you can explore your destination by walking, biking, or hiking, or use the facilities at your hotel, such as the gym, pool, or garden.

- **When you are at work.** Work can be a busy and stressful time for the DASH diet and exercise program, as you may have to deal with deadlines, meetings, and other demands. But you can still follow the DASH diet and exercise program with some strategies and solutions. You can bring your own lunch and snacks or order from a healthy delivery service to avoid the temptation of vending machines, cafeterias, or fast food. You can also keep a water bottle, a tea bag, or a coffee maker at your desk to stay hydrated and energized. For exercise, you can take advantage of your breaks, such as walking, stretching, or climbing stairs, or join a fitness class, a sports team, or a walking group after work or during lunch.

- **When you are at home.** Home can be a comfortable and convenient place for the DASH diet and exercise program, as you have more control and flexibility over your food and activities. But you can also face some challenges, such as boredom, distractions, or temptations. You can overcome these challenges with some tips and tricks. You can stock your pantry, fridge, and freezer with healthy and tasty ingredients, cook your own meals, or try new recipes that follow the DASH diet. You can also involve your family, friends, or pets in your meals, snacks, and physical activities to make them more fun and social. For exercise, you can use your own equipment, such as weights, bands, or mats, or stream online videos, podcasts, or apps that offer a variety of workouts, such as cardio, strength, or yoga.

How to enjoy the DASH diet and exercise program and its lasting effects

The DASH diet and exercise program are not only good for your health but also for your happiness and satisfaction. You can enjoy the DASH diet and exercise program and its lasting effects with some tips and tricks. Here are some ways to enjoy the DASH diet and exercise program and its lasting effects:

- **Appreciate the variety and flavor of the DASH diet.** The DASH diet offers a wide range of foods and beverages that are nutritious and delicious. You can enjoy the variety and flavor of the DASH diet by trying new foods, cuisines, spices, herbs, and sauces that are low in sodium, saturated fat, and added sugars and high in potassium, calcium, magnesium, fiber, and protein. You can also experiment with different cooking methods, such as baking, grilling, steaming, or roasting, that can enhance the taste and texture of your food.
- **Enjoy the benefits of exercise.** Exercise can improve your physical, mental, and emotional

health, as well as your mood, energy, and confidence. You can enjoy the benefits of exercise by noticing how your body feels, looks, and performs after your workout. You can also acknowledge how your mind and emotions are affected by your exercise, such as feeling more relaxed, alert, and positive. You can also celebrate your achievements, such as reaching a new distance, speed, or intensity, or mastering a new skill or technique.

- **Share your experience and results with others.** Sharing your experience and results with others can help you enjoy the DASH diet and exercise program and its lasting effects. You can share your experience and results with others by telling them about your goals, progress, and achievements, and how the DASH diet and exercise program have changed your life. You can also inspire and motivate others to join you or try the DASH diet and exercise program by showing them your results, such as your lower blood pressure, weight, or cholesterol, or your improved fitness, health, or well-being. You can also support and encourage others who are on the DASH diet and exercise program by offering them advice, feedback, or companionship.

CHAPTER 6

How to Make Healthy Food Choices on the DASH Diet and Exercise Program for Special Populations: Adapting to Your Age, Gender, Health Condition, and Lifestyle

The DASH diet and exercise program is a proven and effective way to lower your blood pressure and improve your cardiovascular health. However, you may wonder if the DASH diet and exercise program are suitable for you, especially if you belong to a special population that has different needs, preferences, or challenges. For example, you may have a chronic condition, such as diabetes or kidney disease, that affects your food choices and physical activity. Or you may have a different age, gender, or lifestyle that influences your nutritional requirements and fitness goals.

In this chapter, you will learn how to make healthy food choices on the DASH diet and exercise program for special populations, such as:

Older adults, Women, Men, Children and adolescents, Pregnant and breastfeeding women, People with diabetes, People with chronic kidney disease,People with heart failure, People with celiac, disease or gluten intolerance, People with lactose intolerance,Vegetarians and vegans.

By following these tips and tricks, you will be able to adapt the DASH diet and exercise program to your personal situation and enjoy its benefits without compromising your health, safety, or satisfaction. You will also be able to consult your doctor, dietitian, or trainer for more specific guidance and support.

How to adapt the DASH diet and exercise program to your age, gender, health condition, and lifestyle

The DASH diet and exercise program is not a one-size-fits-all approach. It can be customized to fit your individual factors, such as your age, gender, health condition, and lifestyle. These factors can affect your blood pressure, your risk of developing cardiovascular diseases, and your response to the DASH diet and exercise program. Therefore, it is important to adapt the DASH diet and exercise program to your specific needs and goals while still following the general principles and guidelines of the DASH diet and exercise program.

Here are some general tips on how to adapt the DASH diet and exercise program to your age, gender, health condition, and lifestyle:

- **Age:** As you get older, your blood pressure tends to rise, and your body becomes less efficient at regulating it. You may also experience changes in your metabolism, muscle mass, bone density, and hormone levels, which can affect your nutritional and physical needs. To adapt the DASH diet and exercise program to your age, you may need to adjust your calorie intake, your sodium intake, your calcium intake, and your physical activity level. For example, older adults may need to consume fewer calories, less sodium, more calcium, and more moderate-intensity physical activity than younger adults. You can use online calculators or consult your doctor or dietitian to determine your optimal calorie and nutrient intake based on your age, weight, height, and activity level. You can also use the DASH food pyramid and the DASH serving sizes as a guide to plan your meals and snacks. You can also choose physical activities that are appropriate for your age, fitness level, and health condition, such as walking, swimming, cycling, or gardening. You can also do some strength training and flexibility exercises to maintain your muscle mass and bone health. You can aim for at least 150 minutes of moderate-intensity physical activity per week, 75 minutes of vigorous-intensity physical activity per week, or a combination of both. You can also break up your physical activity into shorter sessions of at least 10 minutes each. You can also monitor your blood pressure regularly and consult your doctor if you notice any changes or symptoms.

- **Gender:** Men and women have different biological and physiological characteristics that can affect their blood pressure, their risk of developing cardiovascular diseases, and their response to the DASH diet and exercise program. For example, men tend to have higher blood pressure and a higher risk of heart attack and stroke than women, especially before menopause. Women tend to have lower blood pressure and a lower risk of heart attack and stroke than men, especially before menopause. However, after menopause, women's blood pressure and risk of heart attack and stroke tend to increase due to the decline in estrogen levels. To adapt the DASH diet and exercise program to your gender, you may need to consider your hormonal changes and cycles, your nutritional and physical needs, and your stress and emotional challenges. For example, men may need to consume more calories, more protein, more iron, and more zinc than women, while women may need to consume more calcium, more folate, more vitamin B6, and more vitamin B12 than men. You can use online calculators or consult your doctor or dietitian to determine your optimal calorie and nutrient intake based on your gender, weight, height, and activity level. You can also use the DASH food pyramid and the DASH serving sizes as a guide to plan your meals and snacks. You can also choose physical activities that are suitable for your gender, fitness level, and health condition, such as jogging, tennis, yoga, or dancing. You can also do some strength training and flexibility exercises to improve your muscle tone and posture. You can aim for at least 150 minutes of moderate-intensity physical activity per week, 75 minutes of vigorous-intensity physical activity per week, or a combination of both. You can also break up your physical activity into shorter sessions of at least 10 minutes each. You can also monitor your blood pressure regularly and consult your doctor if you notice any changes or symptoms. You can also manage your stress and emotions by practicing relaxation techniques such as deep breathing, meditation, or listening to music. You can also seek social support from your family, friends, or professional counselors. You can also celebrate and appreciate the beauty and strength of your gender and respect the diversity and uniqueness of others.

The special considerations and precautions for different groups of people on the DASH diet and exercise program

The DASH diet and exercise program is generally safe and beneficial for most people, but there may be some special considerations and precautions for different groups of people, depending on their health condition, medication, or dietary restriction. Before starting or changing the DASH diet and exercise program, you should always consult your doctor, dietitian, or trainer for professional advice and guidance. You should also monitor your blood pressure, blood sugar, cholesterol, and other health indicators regularly and report any changes or symptoms to your doctor. Here are some examples of special considerations and precautions for different groups of people on the DASH diet and exercise program:

- **People with diabetes:** The DASH diet and exercise program can help people with diabetes lower their blood pressure and improve their blood sugar and insulin levels. However, they may need to be careful about their carbohydrate intake, especially from fruits, dairy products, and grains, as these foods can raise their blood sugar levels. They may also need to adjust their medication or insulin dosage, as the DASH diet and exercise program can lower their blood sugar levels. They should check their blood sugar levels before and after meals and physical activity and follow their doctor's instructions on how to manage their diabetes. They should also avoid foods and drinks that contain added sugar, such as sweets, sodas, and juices, as these can spike their blood sugar levels and increase their calorie intake. They should also limit their alcohol intake, as alcohol can interfere with their blood sugar and insulin levels. They should also drink plenty of water and stay hydrated, as dehydration can affect their blood sugar and insulin levels. They should also eat regular meals and snacks and avoid skipping or delaying them, as this can cause their blood sugar levels to fluctuate. They should also choose foods that are high in fiber, protein, and healthy fats, as these can help them feel full and satisfied and prevent overeating and cravings. They should also include foods that are rich in magnesium, potassium, and chromium, as these minerals can help regulate their blood sugar and insulin levels. Some examples of these foods are nuts, seeds, beans, leafy greens, bananas, and whole grains.

- **People with chronic kidney disease:** The DASH diet and exercise program can help people with chronic kidney disease lower their blood pressure and protect their kidney function. However, they may need to limit their sodium, potassium, phosphorus, and protein intake, as these nutrients can build up in their blood and damage their kidneys. They may also need to limit their fluid intake, as excess fluid can cause swelling, high blood pressure, and heart problems. They should follow their doctor's or dietitian's recommendations on how much sodium, potassium, phosphorus, protein, and fluid they can consume per day and choose foods and drinks that are low in these nutrients. They should also avoid foods and drinks that contain added salt, such as processed foods, canned foods, sauces, dressings, and snacks, as these can increase their sodium intake. They should also avoid foods and drinks that are high in potassium, such as bananas, oranges, tomatoes, potatoes, spinach, and dairy products, as these can increase their potassium intake. They should also avoid foods and drinks that are high in phosphorus, such as cheese, milk, yogurt, nuts, seeds, beans, and cola, as these can increase their phosphorus intake. They should also avoid foods and drinks that are high in protein, such as meat, poultry, fish, eggs, and soy products, as these can increase their protein intake. They should also avoid foods and drinks that are high in fluid, such as soups, juices, and coffee, as these can increase their fluid intake. They should also drink water and other fluids only when they are thirsty, measure their urine output and weight daily, and report any changes to their doctor. They should also eat foods that are high in fiber, antioxidants, and anti-inflammatory compounds, as these can help prevent constipation, oxidative stress, and inflammation, which can worsen their kidney function. Some examples of these foods are fruits, vegetables, whole grains, and olive oil.

How to deal with common issues and challenges for different groups of people on the DASH diet and exercise program

The DASH diet and exercise program can be challenging for some people, especially if they are used to a different way of eating and living. They may face some issues and difficulties, such as cravings, boredom, social pressure, lack of time, lack of resources, or lack of motivation. These issues and challenges can affect their adherence to and success with the DASH diet and exercise program. However, they can be overcome with some strategies and solutions, such as:

-**Cravings:** Cravings are the intense urges to eat or drink something that is not part of the DASH diet and exercise program, such as salty, fatty, or sugary foods and drinks. Cravings can be triggered by various factors, such as hunger, stress, emotions, habits, or memories. To deal with cravings, you can try the following tips:

- Identify the source of your cravings and address them. For example, if you are hungry, eat a healthy snack or meal that is part of the DASH diet and exercise program. If you are stressed, practice some relaxation techniques, such as deep breathing, meditation, or listening to music. If you are emotional, express your feelings to someone you trust or write them down in a journal. If you are habitual, break the cycle by changing your routine or environment. If you are nostalgic, find a healthier alternative that reminds you of the food or drink you crave, such as a fruit salad instead of a candy bar.

- Distract yourself from your cravings by doing something else that is enjoyable and engaging, such as reading, playing, or working on a hobby. You can also call a friend, family member, or support group for some encouragement and distraction.

- Delay your cravings by telling yourself that you will wait for 10 minutes before giving in to them. You can also set a timer or an alarm to remind you of your delay. During this time, you can use the previous tips to distract yourself or address the source of your cravings. You may find that your cravings subside or disappear after the delay.

- Deny your cravings by telling yourself that you do not need or want the food or drink that you crave and that you are better off without it. You can also remind yourself of the benefits of the DASH diet and exercise program and the consequences of giving in to your cravings. You can also use positive affirmations, such as "I am strong and in control of my choices" or "I am proud of myself for sticking to the DASH diet and exercise program.".

- Decide on your cravings by making a conscious and informed choice about whether to indulge or resist them. You can use a pros and cons list to weigh the advantages and disadvantages of each option. You can also use a rating scale to measure the intensity and importance of your cravings and the satisfaction and regret of indulging or resisting them. You can also use a reward system to motivate yourself to resist your cravings, such as giving yourself a treat or a compliment for every craving that you overcome. However, if you decide to indulge your cravings, you should do so in moderation and with mindfulness and not let it derail your overall progress on the DASH diet and exercise program. You should also forgive yourself, move on, and not feel guilty or ashamed of your choice.

-Boredom: Boredom is the feeling of being uninterested or dissatisfied with the DASH diet and exercise program, such as eating the same foods, doing the same exercises, or following the same routine. Boredom can lead to a loss of enthusiasm, motivation, and adherence to the DASH diet and exercise program. To deal with boredom, you can try the following tips:

- Vary your foods and meals by trying new recipes, ingredients, spices, or cuisines that are part of the DASH diet and exercise program. You can also experiment with different combinations, portions, or presentations of your foods and meals. You can also plan your meals ahead of time or use a meal delivery service that offers DASH-friendly options.
- Vary your exercises and activities by trying new types, modes, intensities, or durations of

physical activity that are part of the DASH diet and exercise program. You can also experiment with different settings, equipment, music, or partners for your exercises and activities. You can also join a class, club, or challenge that offers DASH-friendly options.

- Vary your routine and schedule by changing the time, order, or frequency of your DASH diet and exercise program. You can also set short-term and long-term goals and track your progress and achievements on the DASH diet and exercise program. You can also reward yourself for reaching your milestones or celebrate your successes with others who support you on the DASH diet and exercise program.

-**Social pressure:** social pressure is the influence or expectation from others to conform to their norms, values, or behaviors, such as eating or drinking what they offer or joining them in their activities. Social pressure can be positive or negative, depending on whether it supports or hinders your adherence to and success with the DASH diet and exercise program.

To deal with social pressure, you can try the following tips:

- Communicate your goals and preferences to your family, friends, co-workers, or other social contacts who may affect your DASH diet and exercise program. You can also explain the benefits and reasons for your DASH diet and exercise program and ask for their support and understanding. You can also share your challenges and successes on the DASH diet and exercise program and invite them to join you or learn more about it. Negotiate your options and boundaries with your family, friends, co-workers, or other social contacts who may offer or invite you to eat or drink something that is not part of the DASH diet and exercise program or to join them in an activity that is not part of the DASH diet and exercise program. You can also suggest or request alternatives that are part of the DASH diet and exercise program, or decline politely and firmly if you are not comfortable or interested. You can also plan ahead for social situations that may challenge your DASH diet and exercise program, such as bringing your own food or drink or choosing a venue or activity that is DASH-friendly.

- Balance your choices and consequences with your family, friends, co-workers, or other social contacts who may pressure or tempt you to deviate from your DASH diet and exercise program or to skip or reduce your DASH diet and exercise program. You can also weigh the pros and cons of each option and the satisfaction and regret of indulging in or resisting them. You can also use a moderation and mindfulness approach if you decide to deviate from your DASH diet and exercise program and not let it affect your overall progress on the DASH diet and exercise program. You should also forgive yourself, move on, and not feel guilty or ashamed of your choice.

-**Lack of time:** Lack of time is the feeling of not having enough time or opportunity to follow the DASH diet and exercise program, such as preparing or eating healthy meals or doing physical activity. Lack of time can be caused by various factors, such as busy schedules, competing priorities, unexpected events, or procrastination. To deal with a lack of time, you can try the following tips:

- Plan your time and tasks by setting realistic and specific goals and breaking them down into smaller and more manageable steps. You can also use a calendar, planner, or app to schedule your DASH diet and exercise program and to track your progress and achievements. You can also prioritize your most important and urgent tasks and delegate or eliminate the less important or urgent ones. You can also anticipate and prepare for potential obstacles or interruptions and have a backup plan or a contingency plan in case they occur.
- Optimize your time and resources by using shortcuts, tips, or tricks that can save you time or effort on your DASH diet and exercise program. For example, you can use pre-cut, frozen, or canned fruits and vegetables, or ready-made sauces, dressings, or seasonings that are part of the DASH diet

and exercise program. You can also cook in bulk and freeze or refrigerate the leftovers for later use. You can also use online or delivery services that offer DASH-friendly options. You can also do physical activity in short bursts, such as 10 minutes, throughout the day, or combine it with other tasks, such as walking or cycling to work, doing housework, or using the stairs rather than the elevator.

- Make time and opportunities by creating or finding windows of time or opportunity to follow the DASH diet and exercise program, such as waking up earlier, skipping or reducing TV or social media time, or using your lunch break or commute time. You can also make the most of your time or opportunity by focusing on the quality, not the quantity, of your DASH diet and exercise program. You can also use a timer or an alarm to remind you of your DASH diet and exercise program or to limit your distractions or interruptions.

CHAPTER 7

The DASH Diet and Exercise Program for Children and Adolescents: Helping Them Grow Healthy and Happy

Children and adolescents are the future of our society, and their health and well-being are vital for their development and happiness. However, many children and adolescents today face the risk of developing high blood pressure, obesity, diabetes, and other chronic diseases, due to unhealthy eating and physical inactivity habits. These health problems can affect their growth, learning, self-esteem, and quality of life, as well as increase their chances of having heart disease and stroke later in life. The good news is that there is a way to help children and adolescents prevent or treat these health problems, and that is the DASH diet and exercise program. The DASH diet and exercise program is a scientifically proven approach that can lower blood pressure and improve other health indicators, such as cholesterol, blood sugar, and weight, in both adults and children. It is based on eating more fruits, vegetables, whole grains, low-fat dairy products, lean proteins, nuts, seeds, and beans, and less salt, saturated fat, added sugars, and processed foods. It also encourages regular physical activity, such as aerobic, muscle-strengthening, bone-strengthening, and stretching exercises, for at least 60 minutes a day.The DASH diet and exercise program is not only healthy, but also delicious, fun, and easy to follow. It can be adapted to the specific needs and preferences of children and adolescents, based on their age, gender, health condition, and lifestyle. It can also be supported and encouraged by parents, caregivers, teachers, health professionals, and peers, who can play a positive role in influencing their eating and physical activity behaviors. Moreover, it can help children and adolescents deal with the common issues and challenges they may face on the DASH diet and exercise program, such as cravings, boredom, social pressure, lack of time, lack of resources, or lack of motivation.

In this chapter, you will learn more about how to introduce the DASH diet and exercise program to children and adolescents, how to tailor it to their specific needs and preferences, how to support and encourage them on the DASH diet and exercise program, and how to deal with the common issues and challenges they may face on the DASH diet and exercise program. You will also read some success stories and testimonials of children and adolescents who have benefited from the DASH diet and exercise program, and how it has helped them grow healthy and happy.

How to introduce the DASH diet and exercise program to children and adolescents

Introducing the DASH diet and exercise program to children and adolescents can be a challenging task, as they may have different tastes, preferences, habits, and attitudes than adults. They may also face various influences and pressures from their family, friends, school, media, and society, that may affect their eating and physical activity behaviors. Therefore, it is important to use a positive, supportive, and flexible approach when introducing the DASH diet and exercise program to children and adolescents, and to consider their individual needs, interests, and readiness.

Some tips to introduce the DASH diet and exercise program to children and adolescents are:

- Explain the benefits and reasons for the DASH diet and exercise program in a simple and clear way, using examples and stories that are relevant and appealing to them. For example, you can tell them how the DASH diet and exercise program can help them lower their blood pressure, prevent or treat obesity, diabetes, and other health problems, improve their growth, learning, mood, and energy, and protect their heart and brain. You can also use charts, graphs, pictures, or videos to illustrate your points.

- Involve them in the planning and decision-making process of the DASH diet and exercise program, and respect their choices and opinions. For example, you can ask them what fruits, vegetables, grains, dairy products, proteins, nuts, seeds, and beans they like or want to try, and how they want them prepared or served. You can also ask them what physical activities they enjoy or want to do, and how they want to do them. You can also let them choose their own goals and rewards for the DASH diet and exercise program, and help them track their progress and achievements.

- Make the DASH diet and exercise program fun and enjoyable for them, and avoid making it a chore or a punishment. For example, you can use games, puzzles, quizzes, or challenges to teach them about the DASH diet and exercise program, and to motivate them to follow it. You can also use creative and colorful ways to present and serve the DASH-friendly foods and meals, such as making shapes, faces, or patterns with them. You can also use music, dance, or humor to make the physical activities more lively and entertaining for them.

- Provide them with positive feedback and encouragement for the DASH diet and exercise program, and avoid criticizing or nagging them. For example, you can praise them for their efforts and achievements, and celebrate their successes with them. You can also express your confidence and trust in them, and remind them of their strengths and abilities. You can also show them your appreciation and gratitude for their cooperation and participation. You can also model the DASH diet and exercise program for them, and join them in the DASH-friendly foods and meals, and the physical activities.

How to tailor the DASH diet and exercise program to their specific needs and preferences

Children and adolescents have different nutritional and physical activity needs and preferences than adults, depending on their age, gender, health condition, and lifestyle. Therefore, it is important to tailor the DASH diet and exercise program to their specific needs and preferences and to consult with their doctor, nutritionist, or trainer before making any changes.

Some tips to tailor the DASH diet and exercise program to their specific needs and preferences are:

-Adjust the calorie and nutrient intake according to their age, gender, growth, and activity level. For example, younger children may need fewer calories and nutrients than older children or adolescents, and boys may need more calories and nutrients than girls. Children and adolescents who are very active may need more calories and nutrients than those who are less active. Children and adolescents who have certain health conditions, such as diabetes, kidney disease, or food allergies, may need to follow special dietary guidelines or restrictions. You can use the DASH diet calculator to estimate the calorie and nutrient intake for children and adolescents based on their age, gender, height, weight, and activity level.

-Choose the foods and meals that they like or are willing to try, and avoid the foods and meals that they dislike or are allergic to. For example, you can ask them to rate the foods and meals that are part of the DASH diet and exercise program, from 1 (hate it) to 5 (love it), and use the ratings to plan the menu. You can also introduce new foods and meals gradually and pair them with familiar or favorite ones. You can also involve them in the shopping, cooking, and serving of the foods and meals, and let them have some say in what they eat.

-Choose the physical activities that they enjoy or are interested in, and avoid the physical activities that they dislike or are unable to do. For example, you can ask them to rate the physical activities that are part of the DASH diet and exercise program, from 1 (hate it) to 5 (love it), and use the ratings to plan the schedule. You can also introduce new physical activities slowly and mix them with familiar or favorite ones. You can also involve them in the selection, preparation, and execution of the physical activities, and let them have some say in what they do.

How to deal with common issues and challenges for children and adolescents on the DASH diet and exercise program

Some tips to deal with common issues and challenges for children and adolescents on the DASH diet and exercise program are:

-Cravings: Cravings are the intense urges to eat or drink something that is not part of the DASH diet and exercise program, such as salty, fatty, or sugary foods and drinks. Cravings can be triggered by various factors, such as hunger, stress, emotions, habits, or memories. To deal with cravings, you can try the following tips:

- Identify the source of your cravings and address them. For example, if you are hungry, eat a healthy snack or meal that is part of the DASH diet and exercise program. If you are stressed, practice some relaxation techniques, such as deep breathing, meditation, or listening to music. If you are emotional, express your feelings to someone you trust or write them down in a journal. If you are habitual, break the cycle by changing your routine or environment. If you are nostalgic, find a healthier alternative that reminds you of the food or drink you crave, such as a fruit salad instead of a candy bar.

- Distract yourself from your cravings by doing something else that is enjoyable and engaging, such as reading, playing, or working on a hobby. You can also call a friend, family member, or support group for some encouragement and distraction. Delay your cravings by telling yourself that you will wait for 10 minutes before giving in to them. You can also set a timer or an alarm to remind you of your delay. During this time, you can use the previous tips to distract yourself or address the source of your cravings. You may find that your cravings subside or disappear after the delay.

- Delay your cravings by telling yourself that you will wait for 10 minutes before giving in to them. You can also set a timer or an alarm to remind you of your delay. During this time, you can use the previous tips to distract yourself or address the source of your cravings. You may find that your cravings subside or disappear after the delay.

- Deny your cravings by telling yourself that you do not need or want the food or drink that you crave and that you are better off without it. You can also remind yourself of the benefits of the DASH diet and exercise program and the consequences of giving in to your cravings. You can also use positive affirmations, such as "I am strong and in control of my choices" or "I am proud of myself for sticking to the DASH diet and exercise program.".

- Decide on your cravings by making a conscious and informed choice about whether to indulge or resist them. You can use a pros and cons list to weigh the advantages and disadvantages of each option. You can also use a rating scale to measure the intensity and importance of your cravings and the satisfaction and regret of indulging or resisting them. You can also use a reward system to motivate yourself to resist your cravings, such as giving yourself a treat or a compliment for every craving that you overcome. However, if you decide to indulge your cravings, you should do so in moderation and with mindfulness and not let it derail your overall progress on the DASH diet and exercise program. You should also forgive yourself, move on, and not feel guilty or ashamed of your choice.

-Boredom: Boredom is the feeling of being uninterested or dissatisfied with the DASH diet and exercise program, such as eating the same foods, doing the same exercises, or following the same routine. Boredom can lead to a loss of enthusiasm, motivation, and adherence to the DASH diet and exercise program. To deal with boredom, you can try the following tips:

- Vary your foods and meals by trying new recipes, ingredients, spices, or cuisines that are part of the DASH diet and exercise program. You can also experiment with different combinations, portions, or presentations of your foods and meals. You can also plan your meals ahead of time or use a meal delivery service that offers DASH-friendly options.
- Vary your exercises and activities by trying new types, modes, intensities, or durations of physical activity that are part of the DASH

diet and exercise program. You can also experiment with different settings, equipment, music, or partners for your exercises and activities. You can also join a class, club, or challenge that offers DASH-friendly options.

- Vary your routine and schedule by changing the time, order, or frequency of your DASH diet and exercise program. You can also set short-term and long-term goals and track your progress and achievements on the DASH diet and exercise program. You can also reward yourself for reaching your milestones or celebrate your successes with others who support you on the DASH diet and exercise program.

-**Social pressure:** social pressure is the influence or expectation from others to conform to their norms, values, or behaviors, such as eating or drinking what they offer or joining them in their activities. Social pressure can be positive or negative, depending on whether it supports or hinders your adherence to and success with the DASH diet and exercise program. To deal with social pressure, you can try the following tips:

- Communicate your goals and preferences to your family, friends, co-workers, or other social contacts who may affect your DASH diet and exercise program. You can also explain the benefits and reasons for your DASH diet and exercise program and ask for their support and understanding. You can also share your challenges and successes on the DASH diet and exercise program and invite them to join you or learn more about it.

- Negotiate your options and boundaries with your family, friends, co-workers, or other social contacts who may offer or invite you to eat or drink something that is not part of the DASH diet and exercise program or to join them in an activity that is not part of the DASH diet and exercise program. You can also suggest or request alternatives that are part of the DASH diet and exercise program, or decline politely and firmly if you are not comfortable or interested. You can also plan ahead for social situations that may challenge your DASH diet and exercise program, such as bringing your own food or drink or choosing a venue or activity that is DASH-friendly.

- Balance your choices and consequences with your family, friends, co-workers, or other social contacts who may pressure or tempt you to deviate from your DASH diet and exercise program or to skip or reduce your DASH diet and exercise program. You can also weigh the pros and cons of each option and the satisfaction and regret of indulging in or resisting them. You can also use a moderation and mindfulness approach if you decide to deviate from your DASH diet and exercise program and not let it affect your overall progress on the DASH diet and exercise program. You should also forgive yourself, move on, and not feel guilty or ashamed of your choice.

CHAPTER 8

The DASH Diet and Exercise Program for Seniors: Preserving Their Health and Quality of Life

Seniors are the wisdom and experience of our society, and their health and well-being are essential for their happiness and dignity. However, many seniors today suffer from high blood pressure, heart disease, stroke, and other chronic diseases due to aging, genetics, or lifestyle factors. These health problems can affect their mobility, cognition, mood, and independence, as well as increase their risk of disability, frailty, and mortality. The good news is that there is a way to help seniors prevent or manage these health problems, and that is the DASH diet and exercise program.

The DASH diet and exercise program is a scientifically proven approach that can lower blood pressure and improve other health indicators, such as cholesterol, blood sugar, and weight, in both adults and seniors. It is based on eating more fruits, vegetables, whole grains, low-fat dairy products, lean proteins, nuts, seeds, and beans, and less salt, saturated fat, added sugars, and processed foods. It also encourages regular physical activity, such as aerobic, muscle-strengthening, balance, and flexibility exercises, for at least 30 minutes a day, most days of the week.

The DASH diet and exercise program are not only healthy but also delicious, enjoyable, and easy to follow. It can be adjusted to the specific needs and preferences of seniors, based on their age, health condition, and lifestyle. It can also be supported and motivated by their family, friends, health professionals, and community, who can play a positive role in influencing their eating and physical activity behaviors. Moreover, it can help seniors cope with the changes and challenges they may face on the DASH diet and exercise program, such as appetite, taste, digestion, medication, injury, or isolation.

In this chapter, you will learn more about how to adjust the DASH diet and exercise program for seniors, how to address the common health concerns and conditions for seniors on the DASH diet and exercise program, how to help and motivate them on the DASH diet and exercise program, and how to cope with the changes and challenges for seniors on the DASH diet and exercise program. You will also read some success stories and testimonials of seniors who have benefited from the DASH diet and exercise program and how it has helped them preserve their health and quality of life.

How to adjust the DASH diet and exercise program for seniors

Adjusting the DASH diet and exercise program for seniors can be a beneficial and rewarding task, as it can help them lower their blood pressure, prevent or manage their chronic diseases, and improve their health and quality of life. However, it can also be a challenging and complex task, as seniors may have different or special needs and preferences than younger adults. They may also face various barriers and limitations that may affect their eating and physical activity behaviors. Therefore, it is important to use a personalized, flexible, and realistic approach when adjusting the DASH diet and exercise program for seniors and to consult with their doctor, nutritionist, or trainer before making any changes.

Some tips to adjust the DASH diet and exercise program for seniors are:

- Consider their calorie and nutrient needs, which may vary depending on their age, weight, height, activity level, and health condition. For example, seniors may need fewer calories than younger adults but more protein, calcium, vitamin D, and vitamin B12 to maintain their muscle mass, bone health, and immune function. Seniors may also need to limit their sodium, potassium, phosphorus, or fluid intake if they have kidney disease, heart failure, or high blood pressure. You can use the DASH diet calculator to estimate the calorie and nutrient needs of seniors based on their age, weight, height, and activity level.
- Choose foods and meals that are easy to chew, swallow, digest, and absorb, and that are appealing to their taste, smell, and sight. For example, you can choose soft, moist, or pureed foods, such as soups, stews, casseroles, or smoothies, that are part of the DASH diet and exercise program. You can also add herbs, spices, lemon juice, or vinegar to enhance the flavor and aroma of

the foods and meals, and avoid adding salt, sugar, or fat. You can also use bright and contrasting colors to make the foods and meals more attractive and appetizing.

- Choose the physical activities that are safe, comfortable, and enjoyable for them and that are suitable for their fitness level, mobility, and balance. For example, you can choose low-impact, moderate-intensity, and aerobic activities, such as walking, swimming, cycling, or dancing, that are part of the DASH diet and exercise program. You can also choose muscle-strengthening, balance, and flexibility activities, such as lifting light weights, doing chair exercises, or stretching, that are part of the DASH diet and exercise program. You can also use assistive devices, such as canes, walkers, or handrails, to prevent falls and injuries.

How to address the common health concerns and conditions for seniors on the DASH diet and exercise program

Seniors may have some common health concerns and conditions that can affect their eating and physical activity behaviors, such as high blood pressure, heart disease, stroke, diabetes, kidney disease, osteoporosis, arthritis, dementia, and depression. These health problems can cause symptoms, complications, or side effects that may interfere with their ability or willingness to follow the DASH diet and exercise program. Therefore, it is important to address these health concerns and conditions in a comprehensive and holistic way and to work with their health care team to find the best solutions for them.

Some tips to address the common health concerns and conditions for seniors on the DASH diet and exercise program are:

- **High blood pressure:** High blood pressure is a major risk factor for heart disease and stroke and can damage the blood vessels, heart, brain, kidneys, and eyes. The DASH diet and exercise program can help lower blood pressure by reducing salt intake, increasing potassium intake, and promoting weight loss. However, some seniors may also need medication to control their blood pressure, especially if they have other health conditions or risk factors. Therefore, seniors should monitor their blood pressure regularly and follow their doctor's advice on medication, dosage, and timing. They should also avoid foods or drinks that can raise blood pressure, such as alcohol, caffeine, licorice, or decongestants.

- **Heart disease:** Heart disease is the leading cause of death and disability among seniors and can cause chest pain, shortness of breath, palpitations, or fatigue. The DASH diet and exercise program can help prevent or manage heart disease by lowering cholesterol, blood pressure, and inflammation and improving blood flow and oxygen delivery. However, some seniors may also need medication, surgery, or other treatments to treat their heart condition, especially if they have a history of heart attack, angina, or heart failure. Therefore, seniors should follow their doctor's recommendations on medication, dosage, and timing and report any signs or symptoms of worsening heart problems. They should also avoid foods or drinks that can worsen heart disease, such as saturated fat, trans fat, added sugars, or alcohol. Stroke: Stroke is a serious and potentially fatal condition that occurs when the blood supply to the brain is interrupted, causing brain cells to die. The DASH diet and exercise program can help prevent or reduce the risk of stroke by lowering blood pressure, cholesterol, and inflammation and improving blood flow and oxygen delivery. However, some seniors may also need medication, surgery, or other treatments to prevent or treat stroke, especially if they have a history of stroke, transient ischemic attack (TIA), or atrial fibrillation. Therefore, seniors should follow their doctor's instructions on medication, dosage, and timing and seek immediate medical attention if they experience any signs or symptoms of stroke, such as sudden weakness, numbness, confusion, vision loss, or speech difficulty. They should also avoid foods or drinks that can increase the risk of stroke, such as salt, alcohol, or tobacco.

- **Diabetes:** Diabetes is a chronic condition that affects the way the body processes glucose, or sugar, and can lead to high blood sugar levels, which can damage the organs and nerves. The DASH diet and exercise program can help control blood sugar levels by providing a balanced and nutritious diet and promoting weight loss and physical activity. However, some seniors may also need medication, insulin, or other treatments to manage their blood sugar levels, especially if they have type 1 diabetes or type 2 diabetes that is not well controlled by diet and exercise alone. Therefore, seniors should monitor their blood sugar levels regularly and follow their doctor's advice on medication, dosage, and timing. They should also avoid foods or drinks that can spike or drop their blood sugar levels, such as refined carbohydrates, added sugars, or alcohol.
- **Kidney disease:** Kidney disease is a condition that affects the function of the kidneys, which are responsible for filtering the blood and removing waste and excess

fluid from the body. The DASH diet and exercise program can help prevent or slow down the progression of kidney disease by lowering blood pressure, cholesterol, and inflammation and reducing the workload on the kidneys. However, some seniors may also need medication, dialysis, or other treatments to treat their kidney disease, especially if they have advanced kidney failure or end-stage renal disease. Therefore, seniors should follow their doctor's recommendations on medication, dosage, and timing and report any signs or symptoms of worsening kidney problems, such as swelling, fatigue, nausea, or itching. They should also avoid foods or drinks that can harm the kidneys, such as salt, potassium, phosphorus, or protein.

- **Osteoporosis:** Osteoporosis is a condition that causes the bones to become weak and brittle and increases the risk of fractures. The DASH diet and exercise program can help prevent or treat osteoporosis by providing adequate calcium, vitamin D, and protein and stimulating bone growth and strength. However, some seniors may also need medication, supplements, or other treatments to prevent or treat osteoporosis, especially if they have a history of fractures, low bone density, or other risk factors. Therefore, seniors should follow their doctor's advice on medication, dosage, and timing and get regular bone density tests. They should also avoid foods or drinks that can weaken the bones, such as alcohol, caffeine, or soda.

- **Arthritis:** Arthritis is a condition that causes inflammation and pain in the joints and can limit the range of motion and function of the affected areas. The DASH diet and exercise program can help reduce the symptoms and progression of arthritis by lowering inflammation, improving blood flow and oxygen delivery, and maintaining a healthy weight and muscle mass. However, some seniors may also need medication, surgery, or other treatments to relieve their pain and inflammation and improve their joint function, especially if they have severe or disabling arthritis. Therefore, seniors should follow their doctor's recommendations on medication, dosage, and timing and report any signs or symptoms of worsening arthritis, such as swelling, stiffness, or redness. They should also avoid foods or drinks that can aggravate arthritis, such as salt, sugar, or alcohol.

- **Dementia:** Dementia is a condition that affects the brain and causes problems with memory, thinking, and behavior. The DASH diet and exercise program can help prevent or delay the onset of dementia by lowering blood pressure, cholesterol, and inflammation and improving blood flow and oxygen delivery to the brain. However, some seniors may also need medication, therapy, or other treatments to manage their cognitive and behavioral symptoms, especially if they have Alzheimer's disease, vascular dementia, or other types of dementia. Therefore, seniors should follow their doctor's instructions on medication, dosage, and timing and seek professional help if they experience any signs or symptoms of dementia, such as confusion, forgetfulness, or personality changes. They should also avoid foods or drinks that can impair the brain, such as alcohol, tobacco, or drugs.

- **Depression:** Depression is a type of mood disorder characterized by enduring melancholy, hopelessness, and disinterest in day-to-day activities. The DASH diet and exercise program can help improve mood and well-being by providing essential nutrients, hormones, and neurotransmitters and enhancing self-esteem and social interaction. However, some seniors may also need medication, therapy, or other treatments to treat their depression, especially if they have a history of depression, anxiety, or other mental health issues. Therefore, seniors should follow their doctor's advice on medication, dosage, and timing and seek professional help if they experience any signs or symptoms of depression, such as a low mood, a lack of energy, or suicidal thoughts. They should also avoid foods or drinks that can worsen depression, such as alcohol, caffeine, or processed foods.

How to help and motivate seniors on the DASH diet and exercise program

Helping and motivating seniors on the DASH diet and exercise program can be a rewarding and fulfilling task, as it can improve their health and quality of life and strengthen your relationship with them. However, it can also be a difficult and delicate task, as seniors may have different or special needs and preferences than younger adults. They may also face various barriers and limitations that may affect their eating and physical activity behaviors. Therefore, it is important to use a supportive, respectful, and empathetic approach when helping and motivating seniors on the DASH diet and exercise program and to consider their individual needs, interests, and readiness.

Some tips to help and motivate seniors on the DASH diet and exercise program are:

- Educate them about the benefits and reasons for the DASH diet and exercise program in a simple and clear way, using examples and stories that are relevant and meaningful to them. For example, you can tell them how the DASH diet and exercise program can help them lower their blood pressure, prevent or manage their chronic diseases, and improve their mobility, cognition, mood, and independence. You can also use charts, graphs, pictures, or videos to illustrate your points.

- Involve them in the planning and decision-making process of the DASH diet and exercise program, and respect their choices and opinions. For example, you can ask them what foods and meals they like or want to try and how they want them prepared or served. You can also ask them what physical activities they enjoy or want to do and how they want to do them. You can also let them choose their own goals and rewards for the DASH diet and exercise program, and help them track their progress and achievements.

- Make the DASH diet and exercise program fun and enjoyable for them, and avoid making it a chore or a burden. For example, you can use games, puzzles, quizzes, or challenges to teach them about the DASH diet and exercise program and to motivate them to follow it. You can also use creative and colorful ways to present and serve

DASH-friendly foods and meals, such as making shapes, faces, or patterns with them. You can also use music, dance, or humor to make the physical activities more lively and entertaining for them.

- Provide them with positive feedback and encouragement for the DASH diet and exercise program, and avoid criticizing or nagging them. For example, you can praise them for their efforts and achievements and celebrate their successes with them. You can also express your confidence and trust in them, and you can remind them of their strengths and abilities. You can also show them your appreciation and gratitude for their cooperation and participation. You can also model the DASH diet and exercise program for them and join them in the DASH-friendly foods and meals and the physical activities.

- Help them overcome the barriers and limitations that may prevent or hinder them from following the DASH diet and exercise program, and provide them with the support and guidance they need. For example, you can help them find or create opportunities to access or use the resources or facilities that they need or want for the DASH diet and exercise program, such as grocery stores, restaurants, parks, or gyms. You can also help them find or create solutions to the problems or difficulties that they may encounter on the DASH diet and exercise program, such as cravings, boredom, social pressure, lack of time, lack of resources, or lack of motivation. You can also help them cope with the changes and challenges that they may face on the DASH diet and exercise program, such as appetite, taste, digestion, medication, injury, or isolation.

- Connect them with other seniors who are following or interested in the DASH diet and exercise program, and encourage them to share their experiences, tips, and advice. For example, you can introduce them to a friend, family member, or neighbor who is on the DASH diet and exercise program and invite them to join you for a DASH-friendly meal or a physical activity. You can also enroll them in a class, club, or group that offers or supports the DASH diet and exercise program, such as a cooking class, a walking group, or a senior center.

How to cope with the changes and challenges for seniors on the DASH diet and exercise program.

Seniors may experience some changes and challenges as they follow the DASH diet and exercise program, such as changes in their appetite, taste, digestion, medication, injury, or isolation. These changes and challenges can affect their eating and physical activity behaviors and may cause them to feel stressed, anxious, or depressed. Therefore, it is important to cope with these changes and challenges in a positive and healthy way and to seek help when needed.

Some tips to cope with the changes and challenges for seniors on the DASH diet and exercise program are:

-**Appetite:** Seniors may have a decreased appetite due to aging, medication, illness, or dental problems. This can lead to inadequate calorie and nutrient intake and weight loss. To cope with a decreased appetite, seniors can try the following tips:

- Eat smaller and more frequent meals and snacks, rather than three large meals a day.

- Choose foods that are high in calories and nutrients, such as nuts, seeds, cheese, eggs, or peanut butter.
- Drink fluids between meals rather than with meals to avoid filling up too quickly.
- Add flavor and variety to foods and meals, such as by using herbs, spices, lemon juice, or vinegar.
- Stimulate appetite by exercising, socializing, or listening to music before meals.

-**Taste:** Seniors may have a reduced sense of taste due to aging, medication, smoking, or infection. This can affect their enjoyment and satisfaction of foods and meals, as well as their willingness to try new foods. To cope with a reduced sense of taste, seniors can try the following tips:

- Enhance the taste and aroma of foods and meals, such as by using herbs, spices, lemon juice, or vinegar.
- Avoid foods or drinks that can dull the taste buds, such as alcohol, tobacco, or hot beverages.
- Maintain good oral hygiene, such as brushing, flossing, and rinsing the mouth regularly.

- Visit the dentist regularly and treat any dental problems, such as cavities, infections, or dentures.
- Consult the doctor if the loss of taste is severe or persistent, and ask about possible causes or treatments.

-Digestion: Seniors may have slower or impaired digestion due to aging, medication, illness, or surgery. This can cause constipation, diarrhea, gas, bloating, or heartburn. To cope with digestion problems, seniors can try the following tips:
- Eat more fiber-rich foods, such as fruits, vegetables, whole grains, beans, and nuts.
- Drink plenty of fluids, such as water, juice, or tea, to prevent dehydration and ease bowel movements.
- Avoid foods or drinks that can irritate the digestive system, such as spicy, fatty, or fried foods, alcohol, caffeine, or carbonated beverages.
- Eat slowly and chew well, and avoid overeating or skipping meals.
- Exercise regularly, and avoid lying down right after eating.

- Consult the doctor if the digestion problems are severe or persistent, and ask about possible causes or treatments.

-Medication: Seniors may take medication for various health conditions, such as high blood pressure, diabetes, or arthritis. Some medications can interact with the DASH diet and exercise program and affect their blood pressure, blood sugar, or blood clotting. To cope with medication interactions, seniors can try the following tips:

- Follow the doctor's instructions on medication, dosage, and timing, and do not stop, start, or change medication without consulting the doctor.
- Inform the doctor of all the medications, supplements, or herbal remedies that they are taking and ask about possible interactions or side effects.
- Monitor their blood pressure, blood sugar, or blood clotting regularly, and report any changes or abnormalities to the doctor.
- Avoid foods or drinks that can interfere with the medication, such as grapefruit, alcohol, or licorice.

- Store the medication properly, and check the expiration date and label before taking it.

-Injury: Seniors may have a higher risk of injury due to falls, accidents, or overexertion. This can cause pain, inflammation, or immobility and affect their ability or willingness to follow the DASH diet and exercise program. To cope with injury, seniors can try the following tips:

- Prevent injury by wearing appropriate footwear, clothing, and equipment, and by warming up and cooling down before and after physical activity.
- Treat the injury by resting, icing, compressing, and elevating the affected area, and by taking painkillers or anti-inflammatory drugs as prescribed by the doctor.
- Recover from injury by following the doctor's or therapist's advice on rehabilitation and by gradually resuming the DASH diet and exercise program.
- Modify the DASH diet and exercise program according to the type and severity of the injury and by choosing foods and activities that are suitable and safe for them.

- Seek medical attention if the injury is severe or persistent, and ask about possible causes or treatments.

-Isolation: Seniors may feel isolated due to living alone, losing a spouse or a friend, or having limited social contact. This can affect their mental and emotional health, as well as their motivation and adherence to the DASH diet and exercise program. To cope with isolation, seniors can try the following tips:

- Connect with other seniors who are following or interested in the DASH diet and exercise program, and encourage them to share their experiences, tips, and advice.
- Join or visit the resources or facilities that offer or support the DASH diet and exercise program, such as a cooking class, a walking group, or a senior center.
- Seek help from the resources or facilities that can assist or enhance the DASH diet and exercise program, such as health professionals, nutritionists, trainers, or coaches.
- Reach out to family, friends, neighbors, or volunteers who can provide emotional,

practical, or financial support for the DASH diet and exercise program.

- Seek professional help if they experience signs or symptoms of depression, such as a low mood, a lack of energy, or suicidal thoughts.

CONCLUSION

You have reached the end of this book, and hopefully, the beginning of a new and improved lifestyle. In this book, you have learned about the DASH diet and exercise program, a scientifically proven approach that can lower your blood pressure and improve your overall health and well-being.

The DASH diet and exercise program is based on eating more fruits, vegetables, whole grains, low-fat dairy products, lean proteins, nuts, seeds, and beans, and less salt, saturated fat, added sugars, and processed foods. It also encourages regular physical activity, such as aerobic, muscle-strengthening, bone-strengthening, and stretching exercises, for at least 150 minutes a week.

The DASH diet and exercise program is not only healthy, but also delicious, fun, and easy to follow. It can be adapted to your specific needs and preferences, based on your age, gender, health condition, and lifestyle. It can also be supported and encouraged by your family, friends, health professionals, and community, who can play a positive role in influencing your eating and physical activity behaviors.

The DASH diet and exercise program can help you prevent or treat various health problems, such as high blood pressure, heart disease, stroke, diabetes, kidney disease, osteoporosis, arthritis, dementia, and depression. It can also help you improve your growth, learning, mood, energy, and quality of life.

In this book, you have also learned how to deal with the common issues and challenges that you may face on the DASH diet and exercise program, such as cravings, boredom, social pressure, lack of time, lack of resources, or lack of motivation.

Now that you have finished reading this book, what should you do next?

You have to review the book and take notes of the key points and tips that you have learned, set your own goals and rewards for the DASH diet and exercise program, and track your progress and achievements, plan your meals and snacks ahead of time, and use the DASH diet calculator to estimate your calorie and nutrient intake, shop for the DASH-friendly foods and ingredients, and use the DASH diet recipes to prepare and serve them, schedule your physical activities and exercises, and use the DASH diet videos to guide and motivate you, join or visit the DASH diet resources and facilities that offer or support the DASH diet and exercise program, such as libraries, community centers, parks, or gyms.

Also, seek help from the DASH diet health professionals that can assist or enhance the DASH diet and exercise program, such as doctors, nutritionists, trainers, or coaches.

Connect with other DASH diet enthusiasts who are following or interested in the DASH diet and exercise program, and share your experiences, tips, and advice.

By following these steps, you can start and sustain the DASH diet and exercise program, and enjoy its benefits for your health and happiness. Remember, the DASH diet and exercise program is not a temporary fix, but a lifelong commitment. It is not a diet, but a way of living. It is not a challenge, but an opportunity.

So, what are you waiting for? DASH your way to health and happiness today!

www.ingramcontent.com/pod-product-compliance
Lightning Source LLC
Chambersburg PA
CBHW070951260726
48661CB00003B/1223